AUTONOMIC TRIAGE

A HANDBOOK FOR RESPONDERS

NATUREZA GABRIEL

AUTHOR OF THE NEUROBIOLOGY OF CONNECTION

BY NATUREZA GABRIEL

Autonomic Compass

The Neurobiology of Connection

Hearth Science

Restorative Practices of Wellbeing

Keywords: A Field Guide to the Missing Words

So, About that Death Cult you Joined?

The Archeology of Shadows

Sport of Kings

Can't Get Home (Stories)

Destoryer of Empire (Collected Poems 2020–2022)

Origin Stories for Children

AUTONOMIC TRIAGE

NATUREZA GABRIEL

Published by:
Jaguar Imprints
PO Box 567, Nicasio, CA 94946, USA

A CIP record for this book is available from the Library of Congress Cataloging-in-Publication Data

Printed in USA

For Talullah

TABLE OF CONTENTS

PURPOSE OF THIS BOOK

The purpose of this book is quite straightforward. It is to train anyone in a public-facing role who is acting as a first responder to

- read the autonomic landscape of the person you are trying to help so that
- how you interact with them, what you say, and what you do creates a deeper experience of safety in their nervous system
- they are less likely to accumulate trauma
- and so that there is a greater likelihood that your attempts and intention to help them actually make them feel better rather than worse.

When you are interacting with someone who has just passed through an overwhelming experience— whether it is a car accident, or being evacuated, or losing a home, or losing a job, or getting diagnosed with a serious illness— the part of them that is available, attempting to listen to you, understand what is happening, and engage is not their ordinary sense of self. Who you are talking to, in that moment, is not the person they ordinarily experience as a self.

Learning autonomic triage is to learn to read the broad contours of the landscape of the Autonomic Nervous System, which governs the body's survival responses, as they are presenting in realtime. This landscape, which is a sort of deep geology of the human nervous system, should inform all of the decisions you make about how to engage with a person dealing with an overwhelming experience, because everything you say and do will be filtered by them through the lens of the state of their Autonomic Nervous System. It is like a pair of glasses that they cannot take off. If the tint is blue, everything will look blue. If it is red, everything will look red. And the person wearing these glasses that color everything will, in most cases, have no idea that they are wearing glasses at all. If you try to point this out to them, they will have no idea what you are talking about.

You, who are not wearing tinted glasses, will not be seeing a blue or a red world. But if you can really understand the colors and contours of the world they are seeing, you can help them, hopefully, get back a baseline where they can shed those survival-level glasses.

I wrote this book a couple of days after a car wreck that totalled the vehicle I was driving, while I was driving it. I was on a highway in a rainstorm when the car hit a film of water and began to hydroplane. It was an electric vehicle, and it autonomously applied corrective steering that failed to stabilize the vehicle and instead sent it rapidly into a flat spin. It made two complete revolutions, revolving like a helicopter blade, intersected a car in an adjacent lane, then crashed head-on into the concrete median in the center of the highway, obliterating the vehicle's front-end and deploying all the airbags. After this it spun another 270 degrees before coming to rest in the middle of the highway, the cabin filling with the acrid smell of crushed metal and plastic.

Once I had felt my body from inside to make sure everything was intact, I jumped out of the car. A nearby driver had stopped, and was on her cellphone calling 911. The driver of the other vehicle, which my car had hit, staggered out of his car about a hundred feet up the road. It took me a second to get my bearings. I would have stayed in my car a moment longer, after it came to a stop, to catch my breath and find my balance more fully, but I had been afraid it was going to explode, and I wanted to get the fuck away from it. I found myself standing on an elevated section of highway five lanes wide, about a hundred feet above a waterway. It was raining moderately and windy. I was wearing yellow sweatpants, running shoes, and a rain jacket. Pieces of my car were scattered about the highway for a couple of hundred feet.

Once I had made sure the guy in the other car was not seriously injured, and once I understood that the woman calling 911 had not been in the crash, I found myself jumping from one foot to the next, working with the adrenaline that was now coursing through my system. I'm glad I was wearing runnning shoes; they felt matched to the task.

Hundreds of cars had pulled to a stop on the highway as I stood in the rain. It was the kind of accident that brings highway traffic to a complete halt. I tasted the water running down my face, jumped up and down, shook out my hands and arms. I let my body turn slowly through space, I felt the highway under my feet as I watched a fire engine cut a swath through the lines of cars, its red lights catching in the water droplets on my glasses. Every few minutes I had to wipe down my glasses, pretty soon the microfiber cloth in my pocket was saturated.

From the time that the first responders arrived, until the time that I found myself in a towtruck leaving the scene, *not a single one of the actions of any of the first responders– fire or highway patrol– was in any way skillful in responding to my autonomic needs.* Not a single one. It was not until I was in the towtruck with a driver taking me to a tow yard that the driver did something that was autonomically informed. When this happened, my relief was so great it felt like a pressure valve releasing. At the scene of the accident, instead, every single interaction I had with the first responders, had I heeded their instructions, would have made me feel immediately worse.

AT THE SCENE OF THE ACCIDENT, EVERY SINGLE INTERACTION I HAD WITH THE FIRST RESPONDERS, HAD I HEEDED THEIR INSTRUCTIONS, WOULD HAVE MADE ME FEEL WORSE.

I am fairly contrarian to begin with, and I am confident in what I know and do because I have been doing it for thirty years. In this kind of a situation, when people in uniform arrive, there is a power asymmetry. The official representatives, be they police or sherriff or fire or EMTs or Search and Rescue carry a certain authority, which is reinforced by their badges and their official dress, and generally speaking if they tell someone to do something, the person is going to do it. Every single thing they told me to do contradicted the primary autonomic needs of my nervous system, which were to stay present to the energy flowing through my system, and continue to work to metabolize it, to let it continue to move through me so that I did not accumulate it.

When the fire truck arrived, and the fire captain approached me, rather than bothering to look at me, which would have been pretty easy to do, in order to ascertain for himself whether or not I needed medical attention, he just asked me if I wanted a medical evaluation. I'm confident that this is part of a standard operating protocol.

A person who has just gone through an overwhelming experience is, generally speaking, not the best person to decide this. In the midst of a surge of adrenaline, I could have been bleeding heavily (I wasn't, just to be clear) and not even felt this.

My response, in the moment, was, *Absolutely not*. This is not even because it might not have been beneficial to be evaluated. It was because I realized, immediately, that I was going to be asked to sit still while I was evaluated by someone who has less medical training than I do, and that he was going to ask me a whole bunch of questions that would make me think about what had just happened, and examine my bodily sensations, and my body didn't want to do this in that moment at all. And so I waved the examination off, and I'm glad I did.

Most people, I think, would have complied. They would have then submitted to something that contradicted the immediate moment-to-moment needs of their nervous system. Had I submitted to the exam, my body probably would have shifted into shutdown, as the magnitude of the situation settled. It's pretty weird to be getting a medical exam on a firetruck in the middle of the highway as thousands of cars pile up waiting for you, no?

If I was in a state of steam at the moment of the accident, instead of moving back in the direction of liquid water the exam would have turned me into ice. And so to that, *No thank you*.[1]

The CHP officer who then arrived on the scene, in trying to get a statement from me told me sit in the back of his car. At first I complied, but you and I both know that most of the time you are being put in the back of a police car it is not a good thing, and my body didn't like this. He then proceeded to ask me a series of questions that landed on my

1 If I had been bleeding, or bruised, or had a concussion or something, I probably would have responded differently. As it was, there were no surface injuries to my body.

body as though he was trying to get me to say something self-incriminating. I'm not objectively sure that he was, but when someone is in a fight-or-flight state, one of the fundamental purposes of the state is to determine who is with us, and who is against us. The nature of his questions immediately led my body into a sense that he was enemy not friend. Within about five seconds of getting into his car I told him I was getting claustrophobic, and asked him to move out of the way so I could get outside.

At that point, he told me he was simply trying to shelter me from the rain. While I have no doubt that this was true, this intention, which is good, is not the way the directive landed in my nervous system at all. Once I was standing on the highway, once I could move, once I could see around me in both directions, and orient to where I was in space, I was able to answer his questions with clarity. It was much better to stand in the rain than feel trapped in the car.

It occurred to me, after this experience, that no one had ever taught these responders to view their interactions with someone after an accident through the lens of the needs of the autonomic nervous system of the person they were trying to help. Why would they? This is not common knowledge after all. It is largely sequestered to professionals in the somatically-oriented trauma healing professions.

I have helped train EMTs, and they are very capable people. I am extremely grateful to first responders, whose jobs are to move toward events that almost everyone else is trying to get away from as quickly as possible. I am also aware of the tremendous psychological costs that being a first responder can bring. This handbook is for anyone dealing with the public who may find themselves trying to help another person who has just been through something overwhelming.

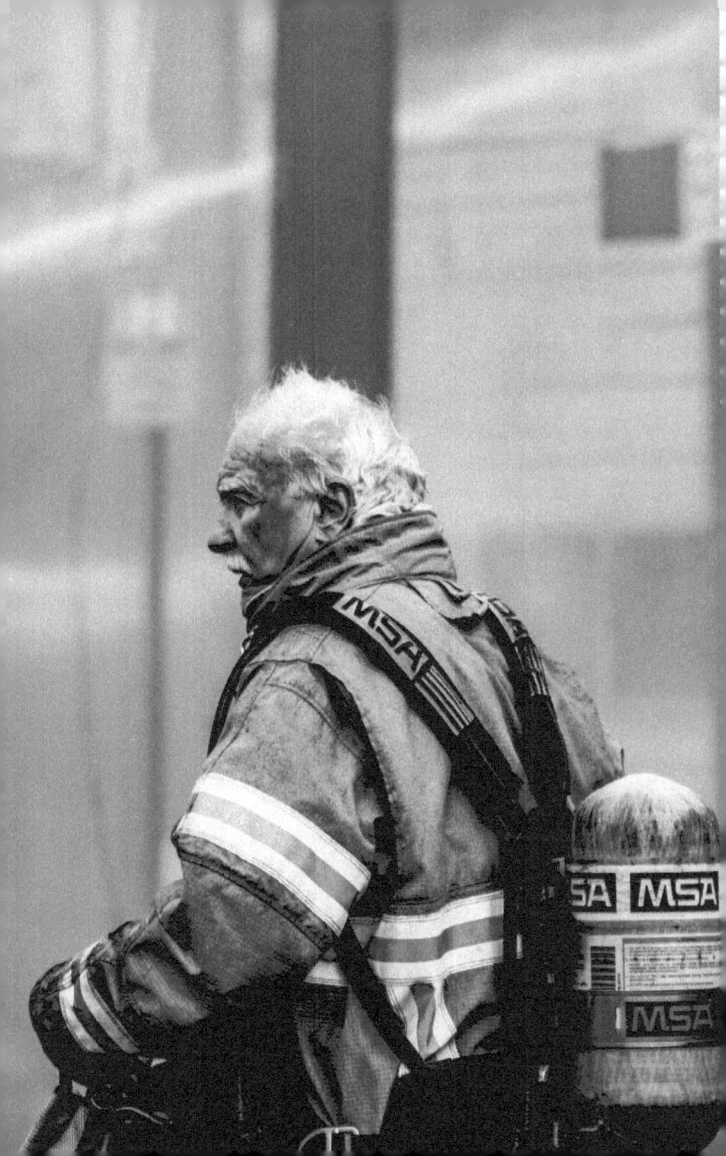

It is designed to help you more effectively help whomever you are responding to, with the added benefit that this is going to help your own nervous system. Because your nervous system, even if trained, is also responding to the social and relational cues of the people you are helping, and if you are not able to read their autonomic nervous systems clearly, you are likely to accumulate vicarious trauma.

All of the triage that you are learning here to help you better serve others you can also apply to yourself. It will help prevent you from getting entangled in other people's survival responses.

You might be a first responder in the general sense of that word, or a volunteer on a CERT[2] team, but you could also be a doctor or a nurse or a teacher, or a coach, or a camp counselor. Or maybe you are just someone who wants to better understand how to support others if you need to respond when someone has an overwhelming experience. Whether someone is overwhelmed because their car just spun out of control 1080 degrees on a highway, or because they just learned they have cancer, or because they got hit in the face with an errant softball pitch, the skills for working with the Autonomic Nervous System are the same.

What I'm going to teach you here is basic autonomic first aid. If you want to go deeper with learning this material, read *Autonomic Compass*, and if you want to go deeper still read *The Neurobiology of Connection*.

Let's do this.

---

2 CERT - Community Emergency Response Team

THE BODY YOU ARE WEARING

Each one of us reading this is so blessed to be wearing a human body. Some wisdom traditions say that the like-lihood of being born into a human body, rather than as a gnat, or a watersnake, or not being born at all, is about as likely as if you cast a life preserver into an ocean, and a sea turtle who decides to come up for air anywhere in the world rises up through the very life preserver you have thrown at that moment. Just to be alive is to win an impossible lottery. We are blessed to be here, even if it is difficult, even if there are moments when it sucks.

Our bodies are one of the most sophisticated instruments in the whole of the known Universe, but most of us have very little idea how to wear them wisely. Their logic is mostly opaque to us. In particular, almost no one in the world understands how the Autonomic Nervous System works. This is ironic because your Autonomic Nervous System is the biological system with the strongest shaping force over our moment-to-moment experience of wellbeing. Learning its language is one of the best investments of time you will ever make. The Autonomic Nervous system, which I will abbreviate as *ANS* in this book, has two primary and related functions.

FUNCTIONS OF THE AUTONOMIC NERVOUS SYSTEM

1) The Autonomic Nervous System governs your internal milieu. It governs the master levers that are responsible for calibrating all of your internal organs and sensory systems in responding to both internal and external environments. In this manner, it governs your breathing, your heartrate,

and your digestion. It governs your body temperature, and how your immune system works, and aspects of memory function. It governs the constriction and dilation of your blood vessels, and the amount of oxygen flowing to muscles. It governs how your eyes and ears and other senses take in information. It governs the tuning of your vocal cords that shape the sound of your voice. It does all of this dynamically, updating with each breath you take. It does this without you having to think about it at all. Wow. Imagine that.

2) The Autonomic Nervous system also – depending on whether you feel safe, in danger, or under lifethreat – surfaces, in each moment, something that I will refer to throughout the book as an Autonomic state.

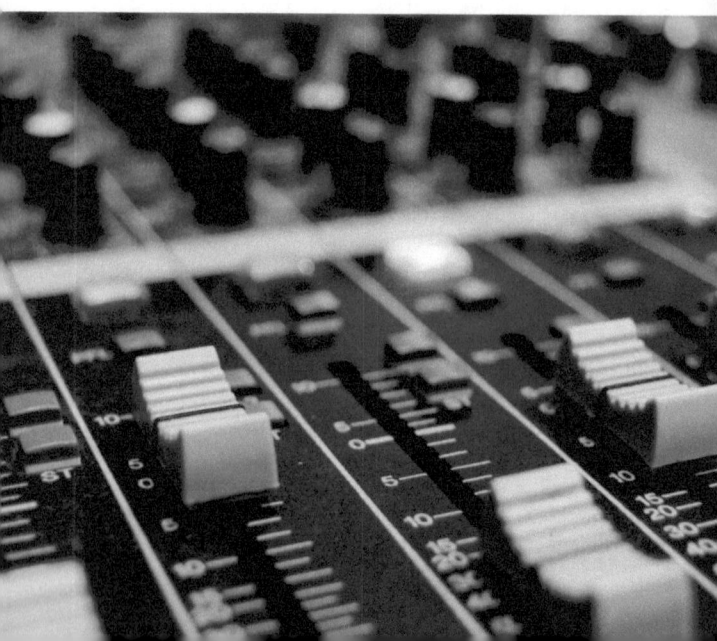

WHAT IS AN AUTONOMIC STATE?

An autonomic state is an energy-processing template. Have you ever been to a recording studio? The sound engineer in the studio's mixing booth listens to the band playing, and adjusts all of the subtle frequencies to obtain the most perfect expression of sound. They turn the bass up, and the treble down, and they fiddle with the mid-ranges. This is what your autonomic nervous system is doing in every moment. It is finding the most perfect expression of sound to respond to your body's assessment of what is happening. The Autonomic Nervous System is the mixing booth of the mindbody connection. It is the sound engineer running your experience of your life, changing the volume knobs on your body and mind.

The Autonomic Nervous System, like a sophisticated stereo, comes with a bunch of presets. These shape the energy and information flowing through our lives. In the same way that you can have a preset that gives you the feeling of an arena in a rock concert, and a different one that feels like an intimate jazz club, your autonomic presets shape your experience precisely. In this manner, the sound engineer doesn't have to improvise each time something happens. They can just find the preset closest to meeting the needs of the situation you encounter. From there they can make micro-adjustments, but the general template for responding is in place very quickly.

The reason that life is so successful is because biology is incredibly good at conserving energy. Our bodies are amazing at tuning our systems very precisely to respond to our survival needs. Most of the time, hopefully, we can run autonomic presets that are pretty low-energy. Most of the time, hopefully, our lives can be somewhat relaxed.

However, if the Autonomic Nervous System determines that we are in danger, or under lifethreat, it will very quickly and severely change the ways that energy and information flow through our mindbody systems. It is capable of accomplishing this transformation of how the bodymind works nearly instantaneously. If you've ever been startled by something, or jumped out of the way of something before you even knew what you were responding to, you have some sense of how quickly the ANS can respond.

These are the circumstances that this book is designed to address. When we are in overwhelming circumstances, the energy-processing templates that the Autonomic Nervous System cues up for us profoundly change the way that we experience our bodies, emotions, thoughts, sense of self, perceptions of the world around us, and how we behave. These changes can happen so fast, and be so extreme, that even the person to whom they are happening has no idea what is going on.

Because the Autonomic Nervous System is the deepest geological strata of the nervous system- its bedrock– it shapes every other system. And what this means is that when a person's body moves into a danger or lifethreat response, and really goes there, this response is going to govern

- their visceral state (how it feels in the body)
- their level of arousal
- their emotional range
- how their thinking works
- how they perceive the world around them
- what actions they take as a result of this

I want you to understand this really concretely. In the moment that our bodies shift from resting states of safety and social engagement into defensive states, such as fight-or-flight, there is a massive sea-change in the way it feels to be in our bodies. This is not abstract at all. Everything both inwardly and outwardly suddenly looks and feels different. When we shift into a fight-or-flight response

- our heart-rate elevates
- our breathing quickens
- our digestion down-regulates
- our eyes lose their ability to see widely and instead focus more narrowly with more intensity
- our hearing changes from prioritizing other people's voices to prioritizing predator signals (think of the musical score for Jaws)
- blood is shunted to our hands if we are going to fight, to our legs if we are going to flee
- it becomes nearly impossible to sit still
- the body begins evaluating our surroundings through the lens of 'who is with me and who is against me'
- the tiny capillaries in the surface of the skin shut down so that if I am cut open by the claws of an animal or a human's knife I will not bleed out
- our auditory processing ability shuts down
- certain aspects of memory function go offline

All of this happens immediately, and without our consent. Our ANS just does this to us. We have little choice in the matter. Once all of these things happen to me, if you are interacting with me you are encountering a person very different from my ordinary sense of self. I will literally feel, sense, see, hear, and perceive things totally differently than I did before this shift happened. What you were saying five minutes ago, that I would have interpreted one way, my body now interprets another way. And I don't realize this about myself.

Learning Autonomic Triage is to learn to read the language of these autonomic states in someone else, so that you can adjust the way that you are interacting with them to help their deep nervous system re-establish a sense of safety and connection, which will bring them back home to their ordinary sense of self. If you are not able to help them do this, and instead they remain in the grip of a defensive survival response, they are likely to experience, feel, think, perceive, and act in ways that continue to escalate their situation, which is not what you, or they, really want.

Learning autonomic triage is to learn how to read someone's state and how to engage with them in such a way that you are providing them the relevant cues of safety and organization such that their nervous system can come out of the heightened states of defense that characterize survival responses. Learning how to do this will make them safer, and it will also make you safer. This is because people who are in the grip of survival responses are unpredictable. They are unpredictable because their nervous systems are reading signals of acute danger. In moments when we are experiencing acute danger, we do not know how we are going to respond. All of a sudden, biting someone's ear off might seem like a necessary thing to do.

Your job is to learn how to collaborate with the needs of this deep nervous system to assist it in coming home to a sense of safety and connection if this is possible. At minimum, you want to make sure you are not increasing signals of danger. You do not want a person whose body is looking for a threat to determine that you, who are attempting to help them, are actually that threat.

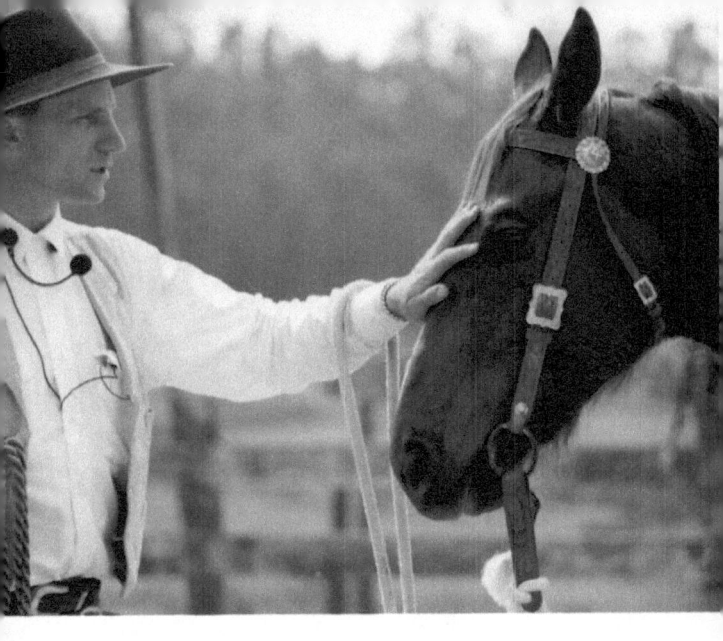

HORSE WHISPERER

It doesn't do a great deal of good to try to talk a horse out of being afraid. Horses don't speak English, to my knowledge. I am pointing this out because in my recent encounter with first responders, I was under the impression that they thought that if they asked me enough of the right questions, in the right order, if they could just get a clear enough picture about how fast I was going, and where the film of water was, and when the spinning started, and where the other car collided with mine, and compile enough facts, they would be able to get an accurate report, they would be doing their jobs, and I would start to feel better about what had happened. This was not so.

The part of my body that needed to be convinced I was safe, after the accident, had, and has, nothing to do with thinking. It is not seeking an intellectual understanding of facts. It is not cognitive at all. The part of myself that needed to settle begins, in fact, where thinking stops. They do not even overlap.

To begin to approach autonomic triage, we have to start to understand that the part of a person that we are trying to reach is not in their heads. It is not the mind. It is not the ordinary sense of self. It is somewhere deeper, and something that can be much more skittish. We are trying to communicate with the body.

And the body is a *feeling animal*.

When we have an overwhelming experience– and people speak about overwhelming experiences in characteristic ways, often calling them *traumatizing*, what we mean is that our feeling animal is overwhelmed. When someone says that something was traumatizing, what they mean is real simple. They mean that something happened, and afterwards their Autonomic Nervous System did not return to its baseline. In the wake of the event they do not feel as they felt before. What we call a traumatic experience is no more and no less than this.

We know when an experience is traumatic for us, because when we revisit it in our minds, it activates arousal in our bodies. There is still an electrical charge attached to it. If you are telling a story about something that happened in the past, but you feel it in your body in the present moment, that's a pretty clear signal that there is still arousal attached to the experience. Any historical experience that can still make your heart beat faster or slow it down just by thinking or talking about it is one that you have not completely metabolized. It is a place where your nervous system has gone up, and not yet come completely back to the ground.

Just to be clear, I'm not talking about *choosing* to enter the feeling of an experience in the past. I can recall certain things that have happened that were pleasurable, and put myself in a bodyset where I can recall viscerally how they felt. That's not what I'm talking about. I'm talking about telling someone a story about an overwhelming event, and noticing that your body, without your consent, experiences the elevation of heartrate, or the constriction of breathing, or other sensations of distress. Those autonomic effects, that you are not seeking out, are a clear indicator of unmetabolized arousal states, what we might ordinarily call trauma.

Furthermore, if you are thinking about an experience that happened in the past, and either 1) you cannot remember parts of it– this happens in accidents sometimes, where there is a part of the experience that is simply not available to your conscious memory, or you cannot organize it into a time sequence, or 2) when you do remember it there is a feeling of the experience being dream-like or surreal that you can still feel in your body, this means that you have unmetabolized shutdown around the experience. I will return to this theme a bit later in the book when we talk about shutdown, but again this is a clear indication that your nervous system went into an ice state, and has not fully returned from it.

I don't know about you, but I have no interest in learning how to live with trauma. Zero interest at all. What I want to understand is how to get people's nervous systems back to that baseline after something overwhelming happens. I want to help them come back home to themselves. I want to condense the steam, thaw the ice, and get you back to liquid water.

But what I want you to understand here, and I'll use the simple analogy of water to explain it, is that if you want to help someone get home in the wake of an overwhelming experience, you have to understand what autonomic template their body turned on to deal with the experience.

SELF AS WATER

Think about it like this. Our ANS is like water. It can exist in three primary states: liquid, steam, or ice.

Our ordinary sense of self, and in fact the place that our wellness resides, is in the liquid water version of ourselves. But sometimes something happens to us that raises the autonomic temperature. If an event gets us autonomically hot enough, we may become steam. Across a particular threshold, the nature of our experience changes. We become a different facet of our autonomic selves: a different energy-processing template takes over. This has very little to do with anything that we choose.

Steam bears no resemblance to water. Once we have become steam, we are no longer in contact with the water version of ourselves. Yet steam allows us to contain and manage energies that are too intense for water. It is therefore necessary and adaptive.

Beyond steam, should it be unable to accomodate the energies released, we have ice. Ice, again bears no resemblance to steam. And yet ice, remarkably, allows us to contain and manage energies that are too intense even for steam. It is therefore necessary and adaptive: a grace.

What I'm saying is the following. If we are going to bring someone back to liquid water, we have to be able to tell, in the present moment, if they have turned into steam or into ice. The difference is crucial. We can warm steam all day long and it will never turn back into water. We can cool ice all day long and it will never turn back to water. We have to know where someone is on the autonomic map so that we can apply the right remedy to get them back home.

And let's be clear: the problem is not steam or ice. If steam or ice didn't exist, you would not be *ok*, because you couldn't have contained the energies you endured without cracking. Steam and ice allow us to change forms so that we can endure overwhelming experience. Steam and ice are not the problem. The problem is when the danger has passed and we cannot get back to liquid water. The problem is when parts of us get enduringly stuck in steam or ice. This is referred to as chronic, toxic, and traumatic stress. The truth is that most people, most of the time, have a lot of themselves stuck across the thresholds of steam and ice. If you are working as a responder, you'll see a lot of this acutely, but most modern people are spending far too much time in steam and ice anyway.

Our job, in autonomic triage, is to help people spend as little time as necessary in defensive survival states.

ITS IN THE NERVOUS SYSTEM, NOT THE EVENT

Here's another crucial thing to notice at the beginning of this learning process. What one person does for fun on weekends is totally overwhelming to someone else. I know some people who would faint if they had to jump out of an airplane, and some who do it for fun. Most of what you do as a first responder someone more cautious might find totally overwhelming.

Something that terrifies one person is thrilling to someone else. And so when we are engaged in autonomic triage it is useless to think about how we personally would have been impacted by a particular event. It is not a useful gauge.

We have to rigorously read the cues coming from the person we are trying to help. Their autonomic nervous system will tell us, reliably, where they are on the autonomic map. We have to have fidelity to an awareness of what their nervous system is telling us.

It is not the event that is important; the question to ask yourself, as a responder, is what autonomic state it surfaced in the person who experienced it. If we understand that, we can figure out how to lead them back home to themselves.

Alright, let's start with diagnostics.

PRIMARY SIGNAL

The first thing I want you to figure out, when you encounter someone who has just been through an overwhelming experience, is their primary autonomic signal.

When I had the accident and jumped out of my car, which I did rapidly because I had the feeling (this was not a thought but rather a bodily awareness) that it might explode, I could not stand still. First I jumped from one foot to the other, then I turned around getting my bearings, then

I paced forward and back. The most difficult moments I had in the immediate aftermath of the wreck were when I could not find my cellphone. My cognition was not working in the way it ordinarily does, but I had enough self-awareness to realize that I needed to get my wallet and my phone out of the car. I had been driving with them on the passenger seat, and when I had hit the median everything had flown around the cabin. The airbag had knocked my glasses off my face; I had found them by fishing around on the ground at my feet. Once I was out of the car, and pretty sure it wasn't going to explode– nothing was on fire– I went around to the passenger door, opened it, and started looking for my wallet and phone. The wallet I found on the floor in front of the passenger seat, but I could not find the phone. This was the most difficult moment, because I was kneeling down, still, *trying to think* through how it might have been thrown, and my thinking mind wasn't working well. I searched under the passenger seat, but it wasn't there. I opened the rear passenger-side door, but it wasn't under the seat. I just couldn't find it. Some part of me knew I would need it to call my wife.

The fact that it was so hard for me to stand still is a very strong indicator of the primary signal here. When we cannot be still, the body is in a fight-or-flight response. Autonomic steam. Its signature is movement energy.

This is the first piece of information that a first responder trained in autonomic triage should have gleaned from me. Again, this is not subtle. I kept jumping up and down like a boxer on the perimeter of the ring. Like I was waiting for my coach to squeeze a water bottle into my lips, and go into the next two minute round. I kept shaking out my hands and my arms, shaking out my legs. This was my body working with the upwelling of energy in my whole system.

I knew this about myself as it was happening.
For whatever reason, even when the car was in a flat spin, I personally did not feel particularly afraid. That is an odd thing to admit, because in retrospect maybe I should have. Perhaps it is because it just happened so fast. The first time I experienced fear, and even then it was not totally lined up, was the moment I felt like the car might explode. That fear got me up and out of the vehicle quickly, yet it was primarily a bodily detection of danger: the cabin had filled with the smell of crushed metal; my animal body was like, *Get me the fuck out of here, that is the smell of war.*

Part of any overwhelming experience is that there is a lot that has happened in a short period of time. Even though the entire accident probably lasted about ten seconds, there is a great deal of information for my body to process and make meaning from. While some of this information is narrative, the bulk of it is sensory and movement-based.

As I stood there, in the aftermath, I kept bringing my attention to my breathing, and to feeling my feet on the pavement. I kept feeling into my sense of balance. My body was shaking. Neurogenically tremoring, to be precise.

This primary signal of movement, of restlessness, technically mobilization, is the opposite of the other primary signal, which is the signal of shutdown.

The signature of that signal is *immobilization*. Someone who is experiencing a shutdown response, which is a lifethreat response, moves into immobilization. Rather than being jumpy, jittery, full of motion, they can appear frozen.

If someone is in a fight-or-flight response, and they are immobilized, they are likely to go into shutdown. If I had

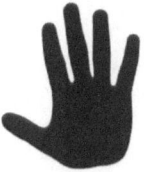

PRIMARY SIGNAL

IS THE PERSON IN LIFETHREAT OR DANGER.
ARE THEY IN A

1) SHUTDOWN RESPONSE
2) FIGHT RESPONSE
OR
3) FLIGHT RESPONSE

ALL OF YOUR SUBSEQUENT DECISIONS
WILL BE BASED ON THIS INITIAL DETERMINATION.

submitted to a medical evaluation, and my movement was supressed, I would have been likely to fall into shutdown. In the back of the highway patrol car, when I started feeling claustrophobic, like the walls were closing in on me, my body was starting to fall into shutdown.

The fight-or-flight state is a danger response, while the shutdown response is a lifethreat response.

While someone in shutdown is more compliant, as a first responder, you do not want the person to go in this direction. If a person goes into shutdown there is a much greater likelihood of post-traumatic stress injury (this is commonly called a disorder, but it is not a disorder. It is an injury.)

If I had complied with the directives given to me by the first responders I would have fallen into shutdown. When this happened, I would have appeared much more calm, but this would have been a lie. Instead, I would have been immobilized inwardly by the release of endogenous opioids. And, three days after the event, I would not be writing this book. I might be in the hospital, or dealing with a host of other post-traumatic symptoms.

If you are responding and encounter someone mobilized this means that their nervous system is closer to shrugging off the event than if they are immobilized. Again, both signals are quite easy to identify if you are looking for them. Yet the intervention pathways for working with these two primary signals are COMPLETELY DIFFERENT.

Everything that will be effective in supporting someone in a fight-or-flight response will make someone in a shut-down response worse. And conversely, everything that will support someone in a shutdown response will be useless for someone in fight-or-flight. So this is the first fork in the road. Until you have clarity about the primary signal, do not proceed.

AUTONOMIC TRIANGLE

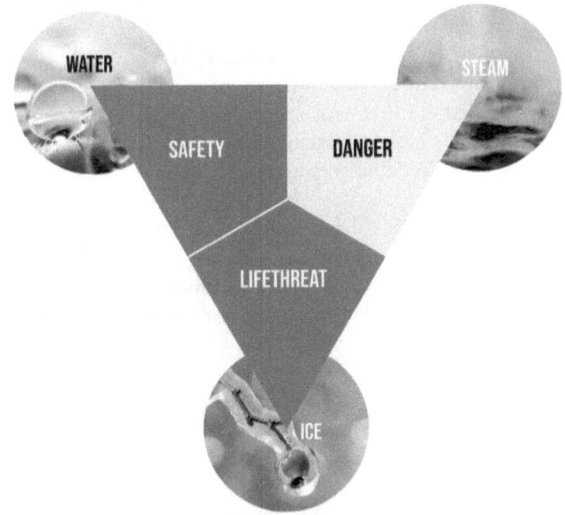

Here are the primary signals: there are three of them. Safety is the liquid water version of self, where wellness resides. Then we have danger, which turns us into steam. And we have lifethreat, which turns us into ice.

What we are going to do next is look at the specific features of lifethreat states (ice), which we refer to as *shutdown* states, and then we will talk about how to triage them. Then we will look at danger states (steam), which come in two primary flavors (fight, and flight) and talk about how to triage them. If you have limited time for study, make sure that you deeply understand the difference between ice and steam states and how to triage them. This is the single most important take-away from this handbook.

There are, in actual fact, at least 12 autonomic states that we commonly see in our work. The map on the facing pages shows all of them on a clock face. Much of our work with people on thriving, on helping people live their best lives, happens in the zone from 7 o'clock to 12 o'clock. One o'clock to three o'clock are danger responses. Four o'clock to six o'clock are lifethreat responses.

This handbook is focused on helping you immediately recognize, and then learn to respond in general ways to the needs of people in the 1 o'clock to 6 o'clock range. This is most of what you will encounter in humans who need your help.

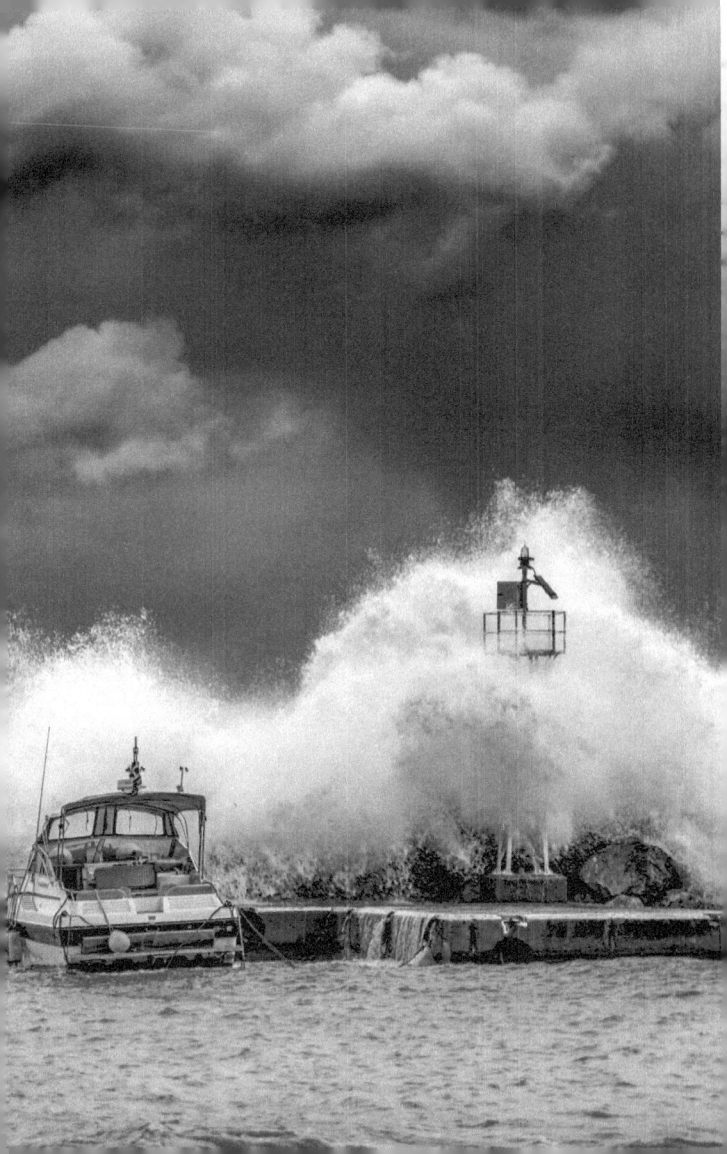

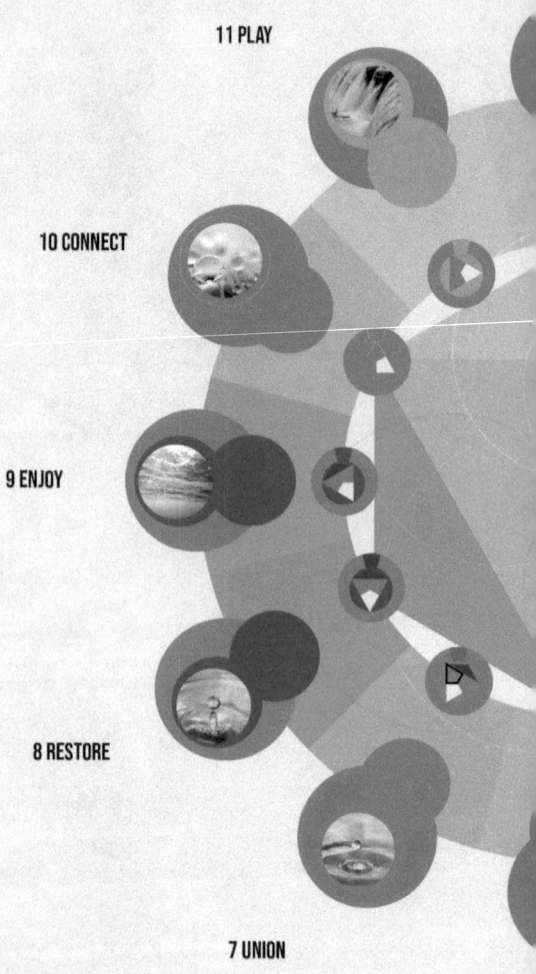

12 COMPETE

11 PLAY

10 CONNECT

9 ENJOY

8 RESTORE

7 UNION

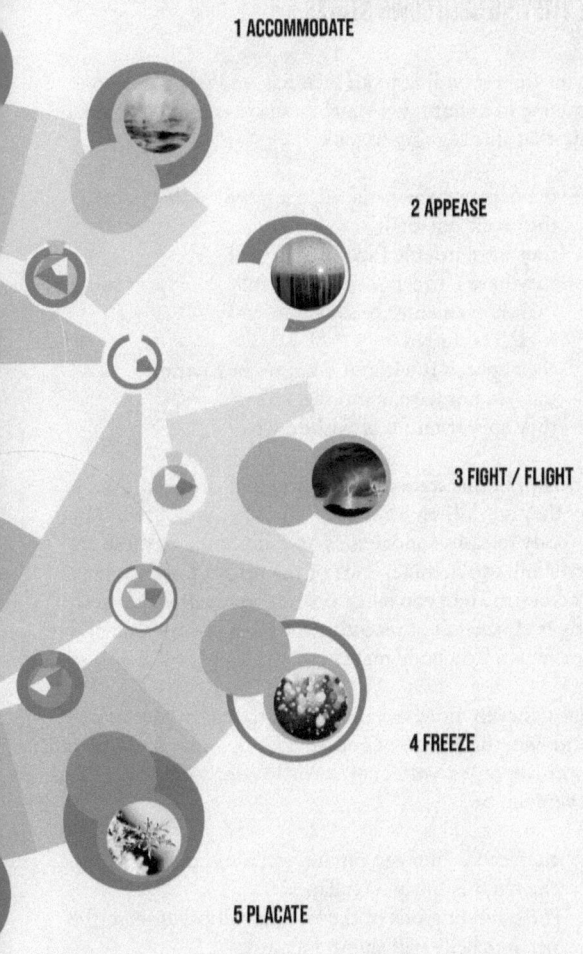

1 ACCOMMODATE

2 APPEASE

3 FIGHT / FLIGHT

4 FREEZE

5 PLACATE

6 SHUTDOWN

IDENTIFYING SHUTDOWN STATES

If you are responding to an incident, and you come upon someone in a shutdown state, these are some characteristic ways that this is going to look

- the person appears dazed, confused, or disoriented
- they look 'out-of-it'
- they have trouble focusing on you
- they have a five-hundred yard state, look past you, etc.
- their movements are slow or clumsy
- speech is slurred
- their speech is without emotion or rhythm
- they do not have emotional affect
- they appear numb or withdrawn

A person in this state can look drunk or drugged. And in a way they are. When we move fully into a shutdown state, the body releases endogenous opioids. Some of these are very similar to heroine. (Part of the reason that heroine is so addictive and people like opioids so much is that your body is chock-full of receptors for these chemicals, because guess what? You body makes its own supply of them.)

Let's get even more specific. When the body goes into shutdown, the release of endogenous opioids blocks certain motor responses, with characteristic effects on posture and movement. So,

- the head is likely to pitch forward on the neck
- the chest is likely to collapse
- the bounding box of the viscera will collapse, so the person's belly will slump forward
- arms will hang limp at the sides

- they will look slouchy

It is the kind of posture that a Pilates instructor or drill sergeant would hate. They would be like, "Stand tall, drop your shoulders, broaden your chest, suck in your belly!" But everything that is happening here posturally is neurological, and under autonomic control, so it is not voluntary.

Shutdown responses are the most severe autonomic response to overwhelm, and they come on strongly when the body is convinced that it is going to die. This means that a person who is really in this state has a body that believes that death is impending. When the body goes into this state, it releases endogenous opioids that immobilize clusters of interneurons in the sympathetic ganglia in the spine, leading to the postural effects noted above.

Oh yeah, if the signal is strong enough, the person may just pass out. So if you come upon someone who has fainted in the wake of an overwhelming experience, and you are clear that they have not been knocked unconscious, you are dealing with shutdown.

You may also encounter another variant of shutdown, which is technically called tonic immobility, where the person is both rigid and immobilized, like a deer in headlights. This is a hybrid of a fight-or-flight state and a shutdown state. We call this a *freeze* state, and will return to it later.

Some other clear indicators of shutdown: if you speak to the person and they
- have trouble responding
- act like they do not understand what you are saying
- do not seem to be able to process questions
- are unable to determine whether or not they are ok

Now, there is some discernment required here, because these symptoms can also happen with someone who has a concussion, or other neurological injury. What I'm recommending is that you become extremely observant. Are they bleeding? Are they bruised? Is there evidence of an impact injury? What other contextual clues can you gain about what happened? Is there anyone else you can talk to nearby who is not in a state like this? This kind of discernment is important because protocols for someone with a concussion, like shining a light in their eyes, will put someone in a shutdown state deeper into shutdown.

What we want to attempt to do, rapidly and precisely, is determine whether the appearance and behaviors we are seeing are a result of an autonomic response or something else. If someone is on drugs or has a concussion, the intervention sequence I'm about to lay out would not be applicable.

TRIAGING ICE (SHUTDOWN)

When you are triaging someone autonomically, whether they are in a lifethreat response or a danger response, the most important thing to keep in mind is that the part of the person that is responding to you is not their ordinary sense of self.

If you think of someone in shutdown as being in an altered animal state– not to in any way reduce their humanity– but rather to keep focused on the fact that you are negotiating with a person's animal and reptilian sensibilities, this can be very helpful.

Shutdown is an overwhelm state. It happens when there is too much information that has entered our systems, and we

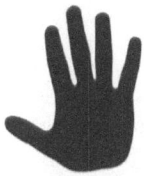

IDENTIFYING SHUTDOWN (ICE)

- DAZED, CONFUSED, DISORIENTED
  - COLLAPSED POSTURE
    - DULL EYES
  - EMOTIONAL NUMBNESS

THIS IS A LIFETHREAT STATE.
ALTHOUGH IT LOOKS INERT, A PERSON GETS HERE
WHEN THEIR BODY BELIEVES IT IS GOING TO DIE.
THERE IS MORE ALLOSTATIC LOAD (STRESS)
BOUND UP IN THIS STATE THAN ANY OTHER.

KEYS TO SUPPORTING:

- MINIMIZE STIMULATION
  - PARALLEL PLAY
- KEEP THEM SAFE WITHOUT MAKING DEMANDS

are unable to process it. This could be information coming in because of something startling, like a person who had just been in an accident where they felt they were going to die. If, in the car accident I had described, my body had reacted as though I was going to die, I had tightened my body, I had been watching through the windshield as the car spun, I had gotten super-dizzy and disoriented, I could have easily gone into shutdown. In that case a significant part of the overwhelm would be unprocessed sensory information. There are also times when what is overwhelming is not sensory, but at a level of meaning. I have trained physicians who deliver terminal diagnoses, and it is very common for someone to immediately go into shutdown when they get news that tests have come back positive and they have a terminal illness. In that case, the overwhelming information is not sensory, but is the meaning. A person can also be overwhelmed by grief at the news of a loss. The response is more likely if a person does not move, or cannot move. If someone screams or moves or reacts in some way motorically to an adverse experience, they are less likely to fall into shutdown. At an autonomic level, wailing in response to the loss of a loved one is a very good idea.

While each of these scenarios presents very different situations, the autonomic result is the same. The person is totally overwhelmed, and their body immobilizes: moves into a lifethreat response.

KEYS FOR SHUTDOWN

When we are working with someone in a shutdown state, the key is to minimize stimulation.

We want to add as little additional information that the

person needs to process as possible. This objective should inform our approach from the moment of engagement. We want to move slowly, we want to keep our distance. We want to speak unnaturally slowly. We want to limit our questions. We don't want to ask the person about how they are doing, because they will not know. Here is how this might look and sound.

I approach slowly and steadily until I can tell the person feels that I am there. I say, "*I. am. Gabriel. I. am. here. to. help.*" Then I wait three seconds.

I make sure the person is not in physical danger. I check for injuries of any kind. I get down to their level so I am not above them. I slowly locate my body parallel to them— the best physical location for supporting someone in a shutdown state is side-by-side with them. If they are sitting on the ground, I sit on the ground, or squat, facing the same direction they are facing. I do not burden them with my attention, or occupy them with needing to respond to me. I get near enough that they notice me, but not so close they need to respond to me.

When someone is in a shutdown state, do not
- Stand over them
- Make direct eye contact with them
- Talk fast
- Ask a bunch of questions
- Display impatience
- Continue speaking
- Move quickly or abruptly
- Touch them
- Expect them to make sense
- Expect them to know how they are doing

It's not worthwhile to give directions or ask questions, because they are not present to what you are saying. Just stop your own momentum. Anything you tell a person in shutdown they will not retain. You are just going to have to say everything again later, so don't waste your breath.

ANYTHING YOU SAY TO A PERSON IN SHUTDOWN THEY WILL NOT RETAIN.

If a person is really in a shutdown state, their boundaries are likely to be very porous. If you touch them they will be forced to metabolize your energy, which can be confusing, overwhelming, or traumatizing for them. They may recoil from touch, or lash out. Ideally, you need to establish bodily trust with a person in this state before you contact their body at all. If you need to make contact with their body to help them or keep them safe, do it at the periphery: hands, or feet. Do not touch their face, their head, their neck, their chest, or their belly. If you have to move someone, try to use their limbs and back to hold them.

For someone in shutdown, eye contact is overwhelming. Speech is hard to follow. Questions are hard to answer. Keep things very simple. If you need to ask questions, make them slow and simple. Ask things in such a way that a person can respond yes or no.

- Did you fall?
- Are you alone?
- Are you warm enough?
- May I put this blanket around you?

Ask permission while recognizing that if the shutdown is deep enough you may be met with blankness. If there are obvious needs, address them slowly, and methodically. Partner with the person if possible. Move smoothly and calmly.

Use your own deep breathing as a metronome to set the pace of your actions. Stay grounded. Shutdown can have a hypnotic effect; so keep in contact with your own visceral sense of self. Keep moving. Wiggle your toes, move your fingers, feel your body.

If you were helping an animal in the wild, and could only communicate your good intentions through the care and quality of your presence, your calmness, and your actions, how would you communicate this intent to the animal? This is how you need to act.

Be gentle and firm. Feel your own feet on the ground. Stay embodied.

If the person begins to shake, and they do not have a concussion or neurological injury, this is likely a neurogenic tremor. DO NOT SUPPRESS THIS RESPONSE. This response is CATEGORICALLY MISDIAGNOSED IN ALLOPATHIC MEDICINE AND TRIAGE.

Neurogenic tremors are the body's innate endogenous and wise responses that allow it to outflow excess energy in the wake of an autonomic shift. If someone begins to tremor in your presense, it means that their body is detecting enough safety to begin to process the event autonomically. This is ice melting. If this happens, do

- stay present and attentive
- encourage them to allow the body to do what it wants to do
- reassure them that what the body is doing is wise
- help them keep their feet on the ground
- the neurobiological center of the shutdown response is in the guts
- it regrounds through the feet

- feet on the floor is helpful for this

You could kindly say, "Ok. So the body is beginning to shake. This is part of how we recover from an overwhelming experience. See if you can just relax and let that happen." Neurogenic tremors may be violent, and they may last for a long time. Do not:

- Tell the person to 'get a grip on themselves'
- Try to stop the tremors
- Grab them by the shoulder or squeeze them
- Tell them to 'Man up' or 'hold it together'
- Try to keep them from moving

Sometimes, as someone has a neurogenic tremor, they will exhibit involuntary or 'ghost' movements. These are related to movement patterns the body wanted to engage, but did not. (Later on we'll talk about a *continuous load path*). Sometimes a person will fight with their body when it wants to move like this, because they do not understand what is happening.

A couple of days after the crash, my body started surfacing the defensive motor movements it would have made if I was not strapped down by a seatbelt. Again, if you see someone fighting with movements that their body is trying to make, you can help normalize them. You can say, "I see that your arms are trying to move, see if you can allow them to do that." You can say, "I know it might not make sense why the body wants to move like this, but see if you can allow it do so anyway."

Again, as a first responder, your allegiance should be to the animal body, not the person's ordinary sense of self, because the animal body is what needs to reset. Since most people are totally unaware of how their autonomic nervous systems work, they will not know that it has these kinds of needs.

Neurogenic tremors can be violent, or they can present as subtle shaking. Often people who are experiencing them do not know what is happening, and this can make them more frightened. They might say, "I'm shaking," or grow morbidly fascinated by watching their body shake. You can help them by saying, "Yes, your body is shaking. This is a natural part of how our bodies recover from overwhelming experience. See if you can relax. It is a good sign that you are recovering. See if you can feel the ground underneath you." Direct the person into visceral contact with gravity.

MOVING ACROSS A THRESHOLD

If you think about our analogy of water, what we are witnessing when someone has a neurogenic tremor, is the melt of ice or the condensation of steam. Their body is moving across an autonomic threshold, endogenous opioids that were immobilizing the body are metabolizing, adrenaline and cortisol are being broken down, they are coming back in the direction of themselves.

Sometimes, if someone is in shutdown when this happens, rather than moving back into liquid water, the person will move into steam. If you observe this happening, it can be alarming. If you've just come upon someone who is in a shutdown state, and they were inert, numb, and non-responsive, and they now come down across that threshold back into steam, they may suddenly begin to behave in a totally different manner. As the shock thaws, they can shift into either terror or rage, the steam state that preceded their movement into the ice of shutdown.

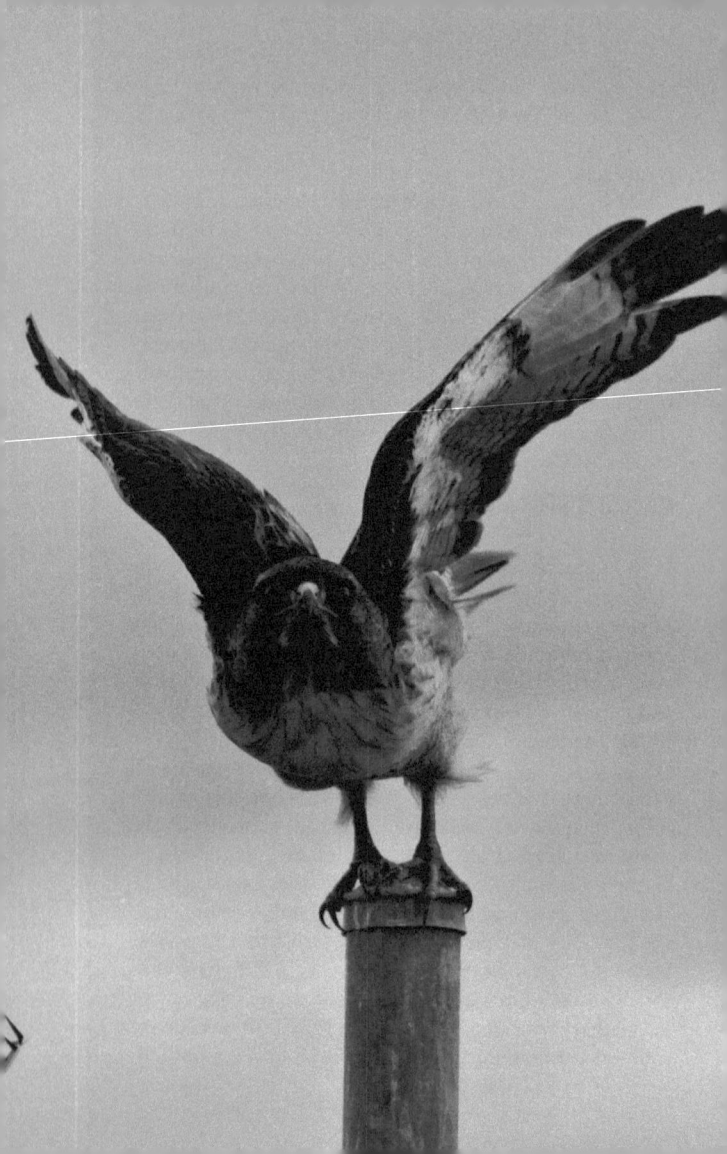

Although this can be very strange to witness, it is both normal, and a movement in the direction of healing. A person in a steam state is in better shape than a person in an ice state. Yet even they might not know this.

When you arrived, eye contact was overwhelming, and so you stayed back. The body then, of its own accord, began to experience enough safety to shift across the threshold. And now, as this happens, the person may turn to you, and suddenly look at you either with rage or terror. You've been sitting right there the whole time, and now this. What you are witnessing is the change of autonomic glasses. You didn't change, but their glasses did. Their world just changed from blue to red. Suddenly they might be staring daggers at you, or looking like they are ready to bolt.

If this happens, you will then move toward triaging steam, which is what we are going to explore next.

IDENTIFYING FIGHT OR FLIGHT STATES

We talk about fight-or-flight states as though fight and flight resemble one another, yet while they have neurology and chemistry in common, the way that they show up in the body is quite different.

Let's begin with what they have in common. The fight/flight states are responses to a detection of danger. In both of them, the neurological system that is most highly engaged is what classical neurology calls the Sympathetic Nervous System. I object to this naming for the simple reason that it conjoins neurology and chemistry that are not always associated, but for the purposes of our discussion here you can just think about it as a sympathetic response.

Fight/flight responses elevate the heart rate. They prepare the body to act. In both the fight and flight variants, there is a release of both adrenaline and cortisol. This is mediated by the hypothalamic pituitary adrenal (HPA) axis. Essentially the response liberates enormous amounts of energy to allow us to either fight off or get away from a threat. Most of us have heard stories about a person who, in the grip of this response, lifts a car off their toddler, or jumps ten feet over crocodiles to reach the safety of a riverbank. In both cases, the performance is a feat that the person could not ordinarily accomplish, yet under the influence of this survival response we can marshall incredible amounts of energy to survive.

In both responses, the primary indicator that the response is active are two features. Both responses are 1) mobilized, and 2) polarized.

FIGHT-FLIGHT RESPONSES ARE MOBILIZED AND POLARIZED.

Mobilization means that the body needs to move. This translates into a level of physical jitteriness that can present as either agitation or anxiety. Like a shark, a person in a fight-or-flight state is never still. The second response common to both is polarization, which essentially means that your nervous system is trying to determine, when there is danger, who is on your side and who is against you. It is a fundamental feature of the biology, in this kind of a defensive state, to see things in terms of 'Us' versus 'Them'. Most modern political ideologies are predicated on this distinction[1], but its origin is psychobiological. If you feel

---

[1]"The best way to bring folks together, is to give them a really good enemy." -The Wizard of Oz, from *Wicked*.

safe, you don't need an enemy. If you're in danger, you need to know specifically who the enemy is. At a biological level, what polarization means is that the body is acutely tracking for affiliation, and antagonism.

Practically speaking, what this means for you as a first responder, is that if someone is in a fight-or-flight state, you want them to perceive you as being on their team. If they perceive you as being in opposition, there is a much greater likelihood of both of you getting hurt.

If you come upon someone and they are in a fight-or-flight state, they may

- having trouble holding still
- may be rapidly scanning the environment
- be talking faster than normal
- be more emphatic
- seem impatient, agitated, irritated, or anxious
- have a lot of emotion
- be bouncing up and down
- want to DO something
- want to take action

It will next be important for you to determine whether they are in a fight response or a flight response. If they are in a flight response, they will

- Be operating on the emotional continuum of fear
- Their legs may be particularly active
- Toes tapping, restless legs, etc.
- Their body language will be evasive
- They may turn away from you
- They will show bodily signals of wanting to run
- They will be scanning for the exits if you are inside

- They may be talking rapidly
- Their faces will show expressions or micro-expressions of fear
- They will interpret your eye contact as threatening
- Their voices will sound fearful, anxious, or nervous
- They may over-react or startle if you move suddenly
- Their thinking will be focused on everything that could go wrong

If someone is in a fight response, they may be

- Confrontational
- Get too close to you
- Have very active hands and arms, i.e., unballing and balling up fists, waving their hands around, putting their hands in your face
- Seem angry, irritated, agitated, or impatient
- Use a lot of profanity and apologize for it if you are in uniform
- Act like everyone is stupid
- Show facial expressions that are large and possibly angry
- Have solid posture
- Move in ways that are threatening
- Make aggressive eye contact
- Grind their teeth and display tension in the jaw
- Fixate on you visually
- Focus their eyes intently on targets (as opposed to flight, which will be scanning for danger)

At a basic body level, if you come across someone in fight it will feel like they might be trying to confront you, if you come across someone in flight, like they may be trying to get away from you.

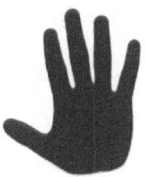

IDENTIFYING FIGHT (STEAM)

- BIG ENERGY
- ACTIVE
- AGGRESSIVE, CONFRONTATIONAL
- ANGRY

THIS IS A DANGER STATE.
IT IS MOBILIZED (NEEDS TO MOVE) &
POLARIZED (WHO IS WITH ME, WHO IS AGAINST ME).

KEYS TO SUPPORTING:

- MAINTAIN ALLIANCE IN LIKES AND DISLIKES
- STAY CONNECTED
- HELP FIND A CONTINOUS LOAD PATHWAY

In both cases, the challenge is to join them, and to get on their side. You need their nervous systems to understand you are with, not against them. The strategies for doing this are quite different.

TRIAGING FIGHT

Take a moment and think about what works for you when someone is trying to calm you down (or support you) when you are angry.

Presented with someone who is angry, we might either feel intimidated or confrontational ourselves. But if you are the angry person, what works to help you lower your fists?

If you are pissed off about something– pick anything...traffic on the way home, the fact that your kid hasn't done his homework again, the fact that your favorite team lost in the playoffs, the fact that your game got rained out– and you express this to your partner, and your partner is like, "Well, that's not very mindful of you. Why don't you take some deep breaths, and then exhale deeply, and then visualize how an Enlightened Being would deal with this," it is likely to make you more angry.

That is because that kind of response, which boils down to telling someone to just calm down, is belittling. It suggests that there is something wrong with the way that you feel, and that if you were just a better person, or more mature, or more evolved, or whatever, you wouldn't feel angry.

But the fight response is about boundary setting. It is about feeling autonomy in our lives, a sense of control, a sense of being able to set limits. And in a world where things feel often out-of-control, where we are surrounded by people taking advantage of systems, and one another, a world that is transactional where it feels like everyone is trying to get over, to exploit every advantage, to screw everyone else, fight is a pretty legitimate response.

I have a lot of respect for the psychobiology of a creature being willing to confront a threat. Small dogs, for example. If you are a chihuahua, there are other members of your species who are ten times your size or more. If there were sixty foot humans walking around, I can tell you for damn sure that I wouldn't walk up to one and bite its ankles, but I've seen a five-pound dog do this to a hundred pound dog. Now, that is really brave. It might also be foolish, but it's hard to deny that it is a courageous thing to do. The fight response is, in fact, one of the most adaptive responses to threat.

The thing that works for me, pretty reliably, in terms of having someone de-escalate my anger, is to have them match my intensity without directing aggression at me.

If I get home, and I'm like, "That f*cking chihuahua came after my ankles again, I'm gonna eat that little f*cker," what I want my fight-triaging anger translator to say is, "YEAH. That's right!"

And if I say, "I'm gonna carve up that dog, cut him into pieces, salt them up, and put him in a soup," I want my anger translator to say, "YEAH. That's right!"

I want them to stay in alliance with me, as long as possible, burning off this steam, until the point where I'm like, "Let's go get the machete."

At that point, I need my anger translator to be like, "No

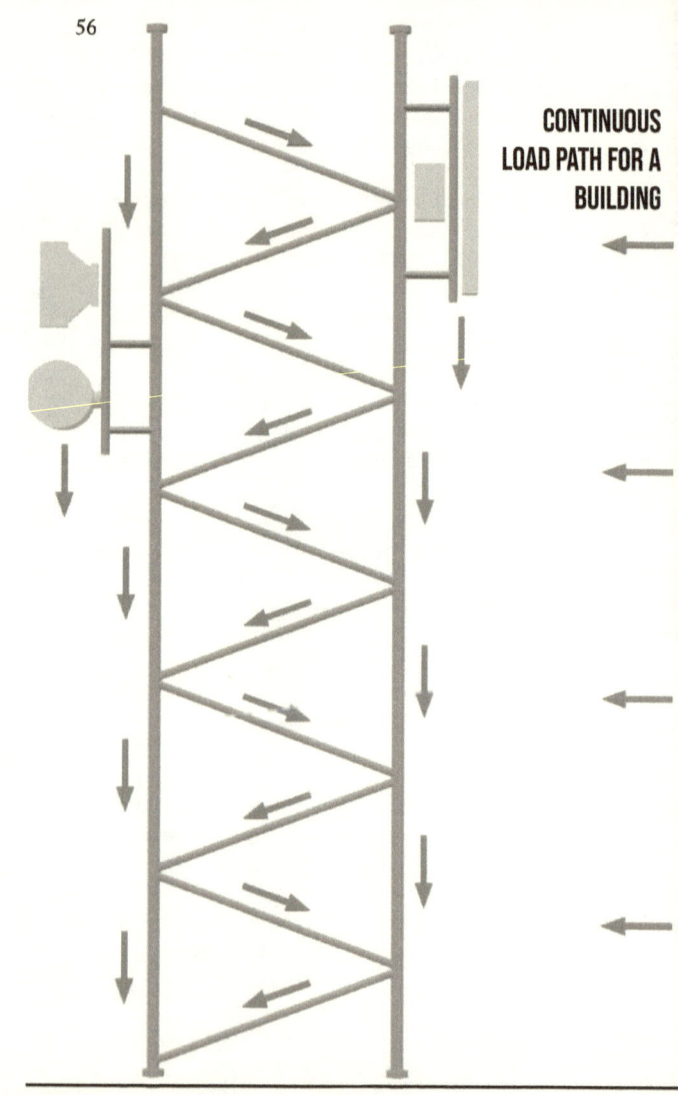

CONTINUOUS LOAD PATH FOR A BUILDING

man, you don't wanna do that. Let's go hit the gym."

My anger translator? At no time were they hungry for chi-huhua soup. At no time were they entertaining the idea of butchering the neighbor's dog. They were staying in alliance with my likes and dislikes, swiveling to stay on the same side of the Us and Them as me.

My anger translator might go home and say, "Yeah, Gabriel is a sick dude, he wanted to eat a chihuhua," – and that would be her right. But what's at stake here is not the ethics of dog-eating. It's my nervous system.

LOAD PATHWAYS

When an earthquake hits a building, seismic waves move through the structure. What modern earthquake engineer-ing does it to give those waves a *continuous load pathway* to move through the building. The load pathway conducts those forces in such a manner that they do not destabilize the building.

In the diagram at left you can see a continuous load pathway for a building being displaced by forces moving from right to left. The load pathway channels these forces in determined ways continuously down the building, from the roof to the ground. If the pathway is not continuous– if it is disrupted at any point, forces will accumulate there and at this point the building is likely to sustain damage, or possibly collapse.

Older buildings do not have load pathways designed into them, and so the concussive waves of a quake can desta-bilize them. High-energy autonomic states are like this. When the body mobilizes in response to an overwhelming event, the body chooses a load pathway to unleash the motor responses of the ANS.

This load pathway is a series of movement responses that are organized by the ANS for self-protection. Think of the inciting event as the earthquake, and the load pathway as the series of bodily movements that the ANS makes to help us respond.

These movement responses are typically coordinated along the central axis of the spine, in Central Pattern Generators in the sympathetic ganglia ranging from the brainstem down the spine in pairs. These Central Pattern Generators (CPGs) are clusters of interneurons that are responsible for generating complex patterned motions of the limbs and spine.[2]

For example– if something flies out at my face while I am jogging, my ANS may detect is visually before my ordinary sense of self realizes what it is, and may send up my arms and hands to block and divert the object as my body twists away from it. With autonomic responses, which you can think of as *automatic responses*, the motor (movement) responses do not travel all the way up the spine to the midbrain dopamine systems for processing, as ordinary voluntary movements do, because this would take too long. Rather, the responses happen in much tighter and more localized reflex arcs closer to the limbs that need to respond.

What this means, practically, is that often by the time the conscious mind registers what is happening, the body has

2 For simplicity, you can think of them as being responsible for limb and spinal movements, but there are also CPGs that govern sucking, swallowing, and vocalization, breathing, digestion, peeing, pooping, and orgasm.

already solved it. By the time I realize that what lurched out in front of me is a startled pigeon, I have already swatted at it and twisted away.

Part of the reason, in elite athletics, that we practice the motion of tennis strokes, or golf swings, or swimming motions thousands and thousands of times is to engrain the motion patterns in autonomic pathways so that they can happen without thought. Athletes are trained to empty their minds, and just allow the body to respond, because this is actually much faster. In working on elite perfor- mance, we learn to allow the body and the ANS to take over and execute movements for us: we aren't thinking about the shots we want to hit.

In the 'earthquake' of an overwhelming experience, the ANS provides its own jolt— the intensity of a survival response— and this endogenous (inwardly-arising) wave of energy powers the continuous load pathway of the move- ment response of the ANS.

The execution of this movement response, and its success- ful completion clears the load of survival energy from the system, and allows us to move back, after the event, into an ordinary arousal state.

The part of us that chooses these continuous load pathways, our autonomic intelligence, if you will, is not our ordinary sense of self. It selects them from a catalog of movement and gesture that contains billions of years of evolutionary history. Sometimes they seem obvious, as in the example where I bat away the errant pigeon, and sometimes it is hard to understand why the ANS surfaces a specific set of movements.

Recently I realized that I needed to move my family. We have been happily living in a townhouse for six years. We own it, we like it, and we were not planning to leave. But a series of events occurred rapidly, over about six weeks, that made it apparent to me, in no uncertain terms, that I needed to get my family out of there.

The moment my body really understood this, I panicked. I remember the moment exactly. It was about 4:30 am, and I was sitting on our couch in the living room, meditating. Everything I was studying inwardly suddenly came together, and I saw with perfect clarity that I needed to help convince my family that we needed to move, and that we needed to do it as fast as possible.

My body, for reasons that are still not clear to me, NEEDED to run around my living room flapping my arms as though I was some kind of flightless bird trying to lift off the ground. The image was as strange to me as it is to you. But here is the interesting thing. This movement pathway that my body had chosen, which made zero sense to my conscious mind, was something that my body itself, my ANS, needed to do.

Until I allowed the body to do it I experienced an almost unendurable level of anxiety. But as I was sitting there, and could not help visualizing this movement, the literal moment that I allowed my body to physically feel the impulse to move like this a wave of nausea overtook me. I went into the bathroom and threw up several times. After which I felt totally different.

Why did I resist the movement? Because I thought it looked stupid. Let's just be real. The movement looked like a toddler having a tantrum. My daughter, when she was about two, and upset, would move her arms around like she was trying to shake them off. I'm almost fifty. I've been socialized to act cool for most of my life, and flailing around the living room like a penguin whose hair was on fire did not pass my test for coolness.

But guess what? My ANS did not care. It required me to execute a precise set of movements: to follow the continuous load pathway it had surfaced. And only when I allowed myself to do this did it re-organize, and did I move from panic and chaos into organized action.

I want us to dwell on this story for a moment, because it is so important. Prior to executing these movements I was overwhelmed, panicked, and increasingly paralyzed by anxiety. As soon as I executed the movements I was able to vomit, and then I shifted directly into a very effective strategic planning mode, and two hours later I had inventoried our entire home for insurance purposes, photographed everything we owned, and put it all into a spreadsheet. In other words, I had transformed that incredible jolt of energy into effective action. Yet in order to do that, I had to execute the movement program.

Let me bring this home for you. Any person you encounter in the midst of an overwhelming experience to which you are responding, who is in either a state of fight, or a state of flight?

They have not yet figured out how to execute the movements of that continuous load pathway.

GETTING OUT OF OUR OWN WAY

When I am training clinicians to support clients in learning to honor their own ANS, I try to help them understand that they don't have to figure out how their client's body wants to respond. The client's body already knows this. What they need to do is help the client *stop suppressing* these movements patterns. We need to get the client's ordinary ego, their ordinary sense of self, out of the way so that the autonomic intelligence can act.

Incomplete motor movement responses get archived in the body as allostatic load. Allostatic load is a fancy word for stress. In the same way that a building without a continuous load pathway accumulates structural stress in components if it cannot dissipate the stress, the human body archives loads that have not found their way out of the body and back into the ground.

The map of where the load pathway has not completed is the same as the map of stress in the body. It is not accidental. If a person has a tension headache, the load pathway is stuck in the head or neck. If they have a stomach ache, the load pathway is stuck there. Frozen shoulder? Load pathway.

The human body has five diaphragms: the thoracic diaphragm, pelvic floor, tongue, thoracic outlet, and tentorium cerebelli. These diaphragms are connected and work together to help move fluids and gases, and to support organ function. Among other places, incomplete load pathways often get stuck in the body's diaphragms.

They often get stuck in the psoas muscle, which is a long spindle-shaped muscle that attaches along the interior of the lumbar vertebrae, and connects to the lesser trochanter of the femur, rooting your leg into your back.

Do you understand what I am saying? If you watch the body closely, it will show you where the load pathway got stuck.

COMPLETION OF MOTOR MOVEMENTS OF DEFENSE

Modern people are socialized in very specific ways. Early on in our development we learn to curb impulses. If everytime I feel in danger and activate a fight response I hit someone in the face, I am getting sent to the Principal's office a lot. If everytime I feel frightened I bolt out of my chair, I don't do very well in school. We talk a lot about impulse control in children, but what we really mean is *impulse suppression*.

And if we are going to share, and get along, and not go around generally terrorizing one another, it is important that we learn not to act out every impulse we have for self-defense. Yet there is intelligence in these impulses, which is something that we often forget in our haste to stamp them out and gain compliance from children.

In overwhelming events, the movement impulses of the body, and their successful completion, are the literal signals whose completion allows us to return to baseline after an event. So learning to listen to, and allow the body to complete these movements is crucial if we want to help people move through and process overwhelming experiences, and not accumulate traumatic stress.

KEYS FOR FIGHT-FLIGHT

If I come upon someone in a fight-or-flight response, it is therefore important that I 1) *respect the body's need to move.*

In my accident scenario, if they had bothered to notice it and understood what it meant, any of the first responders could have seen that I was in a fight response. I was hopping around like a boxer between rounds, and I kept shaking out my arms and my hands. My body was looking for a motherfucker to punch. (I would have liked to punch my fucking car, and in fact the last thing I did before leaving it at the tow yard was exactly this, but I didn't realize that at the time[3]).

Just relating this story I am cursing, and I am allowing this to flow through onto the page. I point this out because it is consistent with showing me that my body was in fight. I don't generally curse in my own private mind unless I'm in a fight response, but in a fight response my inner dialog sounds like it is written by a drunken sailor.

Most of us have been trained not to go into cascades of profanity around people in uniform– that generally doesn't end well– so by the time first responders are arriving, I'm already internally suppressing my autonomic response.

(For fun, let's imagine a dialog with a CHP officer where you didn't suppress this impulse…

California Highway Patrol: *Alright sir, so what exactly happened?*

Unedited me with sailor ANS unleashed: *You see this…blue… Model…3? This navy blue motherfucker right here?*

---

3 When I attempted to steer into the skid, nothing happened. The Tesla's auto-correct function had taken over and nothing I was doing had an effect. The reason I wanted to punch the car? It had stopped doing what I told it to do.

I'm in the center lane doin' about sixty, I hit a patch of water, and this piece of shit with wheels, this fucking robot shitbird, this flighless-automated-fucking-dumbass machine, as it begins to hydroplane, decides to take over autonomously steering the goddam vehicle. Did I ask it to do that? Fuck no. Did it consult with me? Fuck no. Fuck. You. Fucking. Tesla. You techno-fascist 15-year-old South African fuckwit Nazi robot. Every goddam time it auto-corrects, the fishtail gets worse. Whose fucking idea was that? Goddam.

California Highway Patrol: *Uh, sir?*

This is exactly how we are taught **not** to talk. But, had I allowed this to happen, had I un-edited myself and unleashed like this, I can pretty much guarantee you that while I was talking, my body would have loosed a cascade of self-protective movement responses that were the continuous load pathway my body was trying to release. If the first responder had had the wherewithal to notice this, he could have helped me complete my autonomic response and get back to baseline right there at that moment on the spot.

But that's not what happened. Lacking autonomic awareness, each of the first responders tried to get me to stand or sit still, which was exactly the WRONG GODDAM ADVICE.

Sorry, did I raise my voice? Pay attention. This is exactly what you do not want to do with someone in a fight-or-flight state. Getting someone in a fight-or-flight state to sit still may make you, the first responder, more comfortable. But it does not help the person at all. It is much more likely to put their body into a shutdown state, which is more severe. It is much more likely to lock in more severe traumatic injuries.

Because I know– *and knew in the moment*– what my
nervous system needed, I passed up the offer for a medical
evaluation, and I refused to let the CHP officer seat me
inside his car when taking a report. I wasn't simply being
adversarial– I knew that my primary responsibility was to
help my own ANS navigate what had just happened, which
was that the vehicle I was driving had gone into a flat spin
and crashed into a higway median at sixty miles per hour,
obliterating the front of the car.

Most people, I would hazard, would not have refused
an evaluation or refused to sit in the officer's vehicle. In
moments such as this, when first responders in uniform
arrive on the scene, the average person assumes that the
professionals know what they are doing. The average person,
if you ask them to sit still while you give them a medical
evaluation, is going to do it. They are going to comply with
your requests.

And for that reason, as the first responder, your requests
should be autonomically informed.

The most helpful thing you can do, as a first responder,
when someone is in fight-or-flight is to focus on maintaining alliance with the person in distress, and to see if you can
help them identify the movement intelligence with which
the body wishes to respond.

One of the most straightforward ways to do this is to
ask them, if they had a magic wand and could have done
anything in the moment of the thing that happened, what
would they have done. And then, as they answer, watch
their bodies for clues about the continuous flow pathway.

If you see the body shiver, or shake, or make movements

of escape (such as running), or evasive movements (such as twisting away) or movements of self-defense, such as punching, or blocking, help the person notice that they are doing this, and see if you can bring their attention to the sensations of these responses, which will feel really good.

For example:

Let's imagine that I am a first responder, encountering myself in the wake of the car accident. I'll pretend to be the CHP officer arriving on the scene to triage myself.

CHP: *Hey there...are you ok, sir?* (Noticing that the guy is jumping around, puffing big outbreaths, shaking out his arms...)

ME: *Yeah, I'm ok.*

CHP: *Looks like you've had a bit of an accident.*

ME: *Yeah, the car started spinning.*

CHP: *Do you have any injuries that you are aware of?*

ME: (hopping from foot to foot): *No, I'm not bleeding. No cuts. Nothing like that.*

CHP: *I'm noticing that you are moving around quite a bit. I like those workout pants, by the way. I have a pair like that myself. I'm guessing that feels pretty good right now, to jump around.*

ME: *I hadn't thought about it, but yes, my body wants to move.*

CHP: *Makes sense, you've been through a big experience right here. Just allow yourself to do that while we're talking. You can keep moving, I'll just move with you a bit.* (CHP officer starts mirroring back the movement, hopping in place.)

ME: *That was fucking crazy. I hit a patch of water. The car just started spinning.*

CHP: *If you had a magic wand at that moment, and could have done anything, what would you have done?*

ME: *Well, I would have steered the car, but I couldn't because the auto-pilot took over.*

CHP: *Show me with your hands how you would have steered it.*

ME: *I guess like this…*(demonstrates the steering corrections I would have made and begins to shake).

CHP: *That's great. Just let that happen. The shaking is part of your body's natural response; nothing to worry about. It's just coming down from this high energy state.*

ME. *Ok*

CHP: *If you had been able to steer, sounds like you might have been able to keep control of the vehicle.*

ME: *I'm not sure, but I think so.* (Breathing is deepening and returning to normal.)

You get the point. What the first responder is trying to do is maintain alliance with me (I'm in a who-is-with-me, who-is-against-me biological frame.) He does this by

- complimenting my pants, telling me he has a pair
- noticing my movements and recognizing they are meaningful
- accurately noticing they feel good
- mirroring my movements
- actively listening

Each of these things, while small, sends a strong cue of safety and affiliation to my nervous system. He then encourages me to visualize an ideal outcome

- *If you had a magic wand in that moment, what would you have done?*

I respond by realizing (my body knew this but my mind did not) that the continuous load pathway, autonomically, wanted to happen through steering the car. As this movement program executes, my body starts to shake spontaneously, which is the load pathway transferring to the ground. The CHP officer normalizes this:

- *That's great. Just let that happen. The shaking is part of your body's natural response; nothing to worry about. It's just coming down from this high energy state.*

He explains it to me just enough that I don't suppress it, which is probably my natural instinct (e.g., *What's wrong with me? Why am I shaking in front of a police officer? I need to hold it together…*)

The general principles here:

1) Identify the primary signal
2) If fight-or-flight, stay in alliance
3) Observe the body

4) See if you can get the person to evoke the continuous load pathway and then move through it

This is a good thing to practice with colleagues. There is an art to affiliation. It takes practice to learn to affiliate with someone's likes and dislikes in ways that are flexible, yet authentic. You also don't want to be disingenuous. If you say something, it is important that you mean it. When I, as the CHP officer, compliment the pants of Myself, as the person who just had the accident, it is genuinely because I like them. I also have a pair of them, because I'm talking about me. You wouldn't say something like that if it wasn't true. You also wouldn't just, out of the blue, seize on someone's appearance and be like, *Girl, I know you've just been in a wreck, but those earrings are spot-on.* The commenting has to be organic. If you mis-attune to someone when you are trying to create affiliation, it is a bigger miss than if you hadn't said anything at all. You can also attune to someone in many different ways. It can be the cadence of your voice, your gestures, your posture. Simply the degree of respect in your approach. You want to communicate to someone that you are seeing them, that you are meeting them, that you are on their side, that you notice and respect their edges.

TRIAGING FLIGHT

Take a moment and think about what you personally need in order to feel reassured when you are feeling frightened, and want to get away from something.

I haven't indexed too heavily on this, but depending on whether the flavor of steam is fight, or flight, the ANS powers up different sets of muscle groups. This is because, generally speaking, when we are fighting something off we

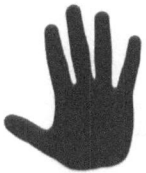

IDENTIFYING FLIGHT (STEAM)

- **BIG ENERGY**
- **ACTIVE**
- **NERVOUS, EVASIVE**
- **FEARFUL**

THIS IS A DANGER STATE.
IT IS MOBILIZED (NEEDS TO MOVE) &
POLARIZED (WHO IS WITH ME, WHO IS AGAINST ME).

KEYS TO SUPPORTING:

- **MAINTAIN ALLIANCE IN LIKES AND DISLIKES**
- **STAY CONNECTED**
- **HELP FIND A CONTINOUS LOAD PATHWAY**

use our front hands, and when we are trying to get away from something we use our back hands (also known as feet). The vertebrate body plan that we are living in undergirds many different types of animals. All of them have two sets of paired appendages. In some of them the front set are arms, in some wings, in some fins. Confrontation typically happens with the front limbs, evasion with the back.

In humans, our hands are also wired into our hearts in unique ways. At a certain point embryonically, the tissue of your hands, face, and heart derives from a common origin.

One of the things that is paradoxical about this in the modern age is that many threats that were concrete ancestrally, as in material and tangible, are now abstract– our ancient autonomic nervous systems don't really know how to deal with the fact that there can be a threat in our phone. We have a really clear deep nervous system template for getting away from a bear. But if that bear shows up in the form of an email or text message on your phone telling you that you are behind on your payments and you could lose your car? Or that the interest rate went up on your adjustable rate mortgage? How do we respond through movements to threats that are abstract? You might run from a bear, but do you run from your phone?

If you are working in first responder situations, however, you will encounter people in flight responses often as a result of concrete events: things that have happened. And if you think about what you personally need to get safe when you feel afraid, it can give you a sense of what someone else might need.

As with fight responses, we want to allow the body to move. We want to find the continuous load pathway. But whereas with fight, these pathways often involve the arms, in flight they will typically involve the feet and legs. Whereas load pathways of fight typically involve turning to face the threat head on, load pathways of flight typically involve turning away from the threat, while making sure that you know where it is behind you.

Doing this involves both the legs and feet, and the eyes and ears. Continuous load pathways for flight make use of the eyes and their intrinsic muscles, the ears and their ability to process predator sounds, and the muscles of the head and neck required to make spatial sense of where a threat is coming from, and to make sure we are getting away from it. Both fight and flight responses also rely on coordination of our vestibular systems, which organize balance, and having a sense of our bodies in space. We need this awareness in order to succesfully confront, and to successfully escape.

CONTEXT MATTERS

We live in a world where safety is not evenly distributed. Where power is differentially distributed, where we are always navigating systems of privilege and oppression. All of us are social beings with social locations: gender, ethnicity, class, age, religion, geography, occupation, etc.

Most of us have experienced harm from other humans, and most of us have harmed other humans.

I like to camp. I have spent a lot of nights sleeping outside by choice. If left to my own devices, I prefer not to sleep in a tent. I'll hang a hammock between two trees, or sleep on a platform. I used to even sleep on the ground, until I once awoke in the middle of the night to the sound of a creature walking onto my tarp, slowly lifted up my face from the pillow, and watched the white line of a skunk's back pass a couple of inches under my nose on a moonless night.

My wife, however, prefers to sleep in a tent. The way I see it, I would rather see what is happening around me. If there is a bear in the woods, I would like to see him first. As far as I can tell, if an animal is intent on eating me, the tent provides no protection. It is like the foil wrapper on a burrito. I would rather see what is coming and be able to fight it off than be tangled in mesh. But happy wife, happy life, right? When we go camping together, we sleep in the tent. Now, the reason I'm telling you this story is because there are sometimes when my wife will shake me awake in the middle of the night, God bless her, whispering, "What's that noise?" in my ear.

There have been times when it has been a raccoon (sounds like a bear), a mouse (sounds like a raccoon), insects (sounds like a mouse), a coyote (sounds like a coyote). If you are frightened, the creature seems much larger.

Raccoons can make a fuck-ton of noise, but they are not particularly dangerous. But if you are my wife, and you are nervous anyway, surrounded by unfamiliar sounds, smells, and movements, the sound of the raccoon gets larger and larger, because attention potentiates experience, until she is convinced that there is a bear, and she wakes me up.

In my ear she hisses, "What's that noise?"
Foggily I say, "It's a raccoon."
She says, "It's a bear."
I say, "It is not a bear."

I reach for a headlamp, and usually turning it on is enough to cause the raccoon to wander off. Sometimes, we open the tent flap and stare at their bandit faces, and I admire their little articulate hands. Generally speaking, these animal noises do not bother me at all. They do not even make me nervous. Unless... the sound is a human voice.

If we are camping and went to sleep in an area where there are no other people, and I am awakened during the night by the sound of strange human voices? Well, Annie get your gun, now I am fucking awake. My deeply ancestral nervous system knows that humans are the most dangerous and unpredictable animals that there are. What I do not want to encounter in the middle of the night in the backcountry is a strange set of humans. Bears? Coyotes? Foxes? Deer? Badgers? Raccoons? No problem. Homo Sapiens? No thank you.

All of this is to say that if you are reading this, and you are a first responder, someone in a flight response may feel the same way about you as I feel about people I don't know outside of my tent. Your mere presence may put them on high alert.

Being in an official capacity (wearing a badge, uniform, etc.) can sometimes be enough reassurance that we do not have ill-intent, but if a person is deep enough in a flight response (or a fight response, or a shutdown response) these cues and clues may not register. What I am pointing toward here is awareness of your own social location, as a first responder, and how it might be interpreted by a frightened animal in a flight state who has been hurt by other humans that might in some way resemble you.

So, for example, the simple fact that I am a man responding to an event could, if the person in distress is a woman who has been harmed by men in the past, cause a woman in a flight response to become more frightened. If I am, as a white man, responding to a black man who has had negative experiences with white men (and find me a black man who has not), the simple fact that I am a white man might make a black man feel more nervous.

If I am responding to a dangerous situation, and my presence makes him feel more in danger, and I can feel that he feels more in danger, and he can feel that I can feel that my presence makes him feel more in danger, we are escalating, not moving toward more safety.

Is this overtly because of something I have done? No. And yet, autonomically, that does not matter. Sometimes maybe I am the only person responding, but what I'd like you to consider is that the more diversity you have in a team of responders, the more strategic you can be about supporting the needs of different groups of people in different kinds of defensive states requiring different kinds of affiliation.

Through developing our ability to connect skillfully with others, we can bridge a lot of differences. But context is really important because in these interactions we are responding to subtle and animal cues, and animal detection of danger. The bodies we are wearing have been harmed by other bodies, and this is part of our survival calculus, like it or not.

Populations with less structural privilege— e.g., women, People of Culture, Indigenous people, people from other countries, people whose first language is not English, are more likely to have histories of negative encounters with people from dominant social groups, e.g., White, male, christian, etc.

Previous interactions condition our autonomic responses. If we set aside our own egos, and recognize that responding is a role of service, we want to try to be sensitive to who is going to have the greatest success communicating a felt sense of safety to someone we are trying to help. It may be someone who shares some cultural background with the person needing assistance. It may be someone who shares their gender, or their language.

What I am advocating for here is that you recognize that sociological categories intersect with our experience of safety, danger, and lifethreat in very fundamental ways. Since our objective is to help people feel safer at an embodied level, this has to be part of our calculus of affiliation.

This has nothing to do with politics, and it has nothing to do with what people think. This has to do with the reality of body supremacy, and that autonomics and culture are intertwined. I would be remiss if I didn't recommend that you reflect on how your specific social location, your gender, race, age, sexual orientation, class, religion, and geography are likely to be interpreted by people you are seeking to help in various defensive responses.

This can help you be less surprised if and when you do not get a response you were hoping for, or if it is harder to get into alliance with someone than you had anticipated.

KEYS FOR FLIGHT

At the level of embodied communication, my objective as a responder to someone in flight is to communicate that they are safe, and that I have their back.

With me, they are safe enough to do what they need to do. Sometimes this is simply to be able to realize that the situation is now in the past, and to take a deep breathe. Sometimes this deep breath is followed by a need to release emotion. To let go, and weep, or express other emotions.

Let's have the humility, as first responders, to be human with people, and to be present for the big emotions that may show up in the wake of these events.

Let's learn to allow our own big emotions to move through us, so that we give people we are serving permission to move through their own big emotions.

Let's not shy away from the moments where someone might need to rest against us, or cry on our shoulder. And let's also not take it personally if someone doesn't feel safe enough with us to do that, and instead find them someone with whom they can.

I never worry about people who are crying in an emergency situation. Crying is sign of health; a sign of resilience. No one gets injured from weeping too much.

I worry about the people who can't cry, because those are the ones simply accumulating the load.

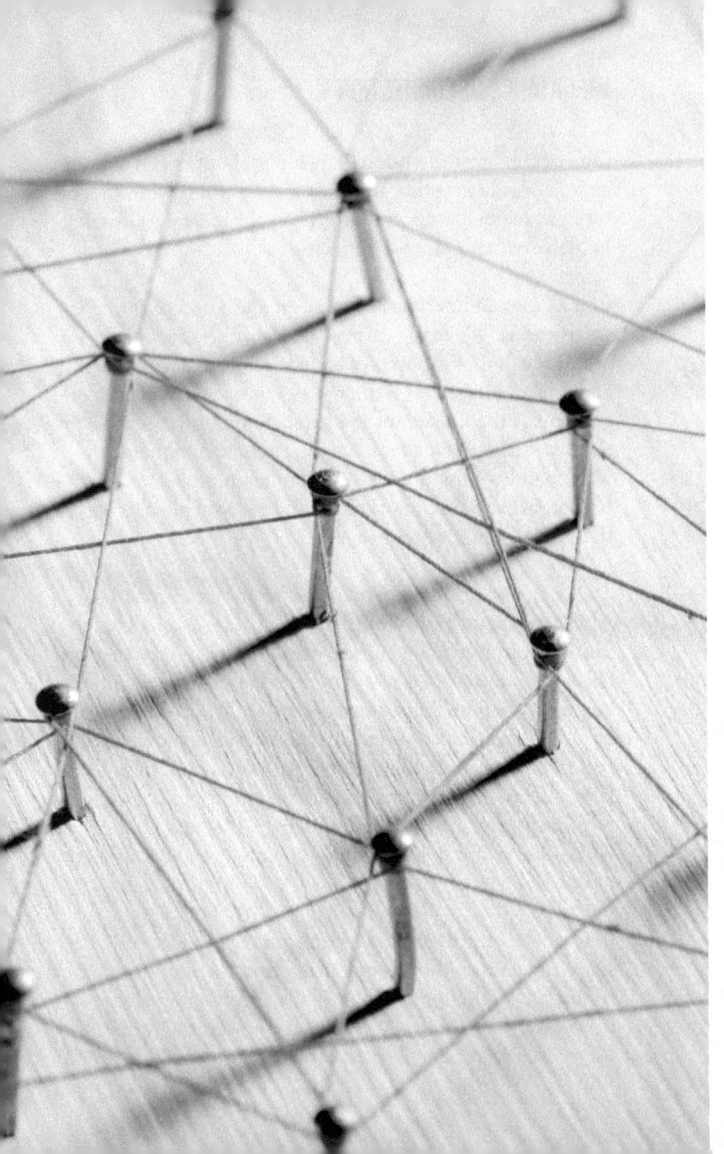

IMPORTANCE OF CONNECTION

One of the most disconcerting things about overwhelming experiences is that they make us feel so alone. Modern culture has really lost touch with the evolutionary reality that human wellbeing is social in nature.

Our bodies and nervous systems are designed to thrive in small bands. We really do need one another. Part of the grand illusion of modernity is that we could accumulate enough resources (get rich enough) to not need other people. This is the illusion of the gated community. Yet when shit hits the fan, what you need are fellow members of a small band willing to help one another, not piles of coin. Reciprocal social relationships will keep you alive in ways that no amount of money will.

The deep evolutionary baseline of our species is one in which we spent 99% of our lineage history in small bands. Think about times in your life when you were thriving, and they often correspond to having a small band to which you belong. Whether this was extended family, a team of some kind, a workgroup, a social club, a spiritual community, or some other place that you felt that you could fully be yourself, and experienced an authentic sense of belonging, our flourishing is connected to being social and connected with others. Our connectedness is literally the living fabric of our wellbeing.

One of the important and unexpected byproducts of surviving community emergencies, from natural disasters to the COVID-19 pandemic, is that in an emergency people are forced to recognize that we need eachother. In these situations people often come to one another's aid in ways that would seem quite out-of-the-ordinary in our modern world, but that simply emerge from the wellspring of our humanity. We share meals with strangers, gather in community, circle up around the fire. Imagine how much better the world would be if we could simply turn on this sense of community care and take care of eachother without needing a disaster to bring us together? It would change literally everything.

Overwhelming experiences are difficult by definition, but they are made worse by the fact that most of us feel alone in our experiences. Because the territory of these experiences is unfamiliar, and frightening, it is very easy for us to feel adrift, and disconnected, isolated, and alone.

First responders are uniquely positioned to alleviate this sense of loneliness because, let's just be honest about this, you have more experience than most people navigating through experiences that other people find overwhelming. By being a first responder, you have likely self-selected for this kind of work, and you are probably a bit of a natural at it.

This is a real skillset, and puts you in a good position to help communicate to people— not simply in words, but with the quality of your attention, how you are present, your own gestures, posture, tone of voice, and kindess— that they are not alone.

I don't know if you've ever watched a young child on a playground take a spill and look back at their parent for reassurance. The kid is like – *I'm not sure what just happened, and I'm not sure I'm ok: what do you think?* Children will take their cues, to a remarkable degree, from the parents. If a child scrapes a knee, turns to the parent, and the parent looks shocked and horrified, rushes in, scoops up the kid, and starts to speak in an agitated fashion, fawning over them, the child will burst into tears. If on the other hand, the parent calmly makes eye contact with the child, holds them with their eyes, acknowledges the situation but doesn't make any fuss over it, maybe just brushes the child off, often the kid will go right back to playing.

Most people are, in overwhelming situations, kind of like the child. You, as a responder, are kind of like the parent. The tools of autonomic triage are the lens that you can look through, at the child, to determine how best to meet their deepest needs. Autonomic fluency, in this regard, is to figure out how to meet the needs of the child (by which I mean the person who is overwhelmed) in a way that helps their nervous system not feel alone.

Throughout this handbook, we have been exploring ways to do this. But what I want to end by reminding you is that in order to fully come home to themselves, what people need to be reminded of is their sense of connection. This sense of connection can be to their families, their communities, to Nature, to a Higher Power. The meta-communication that we want to give people, by which I mean the over-arching impression we want to leave them with, in the wake of being with us, is that we care about them, they are seen, they matter, and that they are going to be ok. If you can help connect them back to this sense, and help them maintain it, it dramatically increases the chances that this will be true.

Because the ANS literally governs the master controls of the body, including heartrate, breathing, digestion, immune function, the dilation and contraction of blood vessels, etc., what the autonomic nervous system believes to be true about a situation often becomes true. If someone remains convinced that they are going to die, which is the primary communication of a lifethreat response– guess what? They might.

WHAT THE AUTONOMIC NERVOUS SYSTEM BELIEVES TO BE TRUE ABOUT A SITUATION OFTEN BECOMES TRUE

I have seen effective autonomic triage where a first respond-er (myself) was able to keep someone bleeding profusely so calm that they were able to be transported to a hospital and bandaged up quickly and efficiently, losing only a little bit of blood. This autonomic triage, which kept the person feeling calm and connected (I can assure you the first responder, who was maintaining pressure on the patient's wound while driving rapidly to the hospital and trying to figure out with the patient's mother on the phone where the patient's insurance card was, was not feeling all that calm) kept sending signals to the injured person's nervous system that said - *Hey, you are gonna be ok. We are gonna be ok.* In those moments, I made it my entire focus to keep sending signals to the injured person (my daughter) that what was happening was routine, no big deal, not a problem.

Had those signals failed, and her ANS gone into a fight-or-flight response, her heartrate would have elevated, adren-aline and cortisol would have been released dilating blood vessels in the skeletal muscles, which would have dramati-cally increased the bleeding. She would have noticed this, it would have freaked her out further, and created a negative feedback loop.

As responders our ability to accurately assess the situation autonomically, to understand the specific needs of states (ice and steam; shutdown, fight, and flight) allows us to focus our efforts on meeting the most pressing needs of the deepest part of the nervous system of the person we are trying to help. This allows us to meet them, to be present with them, and to come through the experience with them. And in this way, we get through overwhelming experiences together.

GETTING ON WITH YOUR LIFE

Getting through the autonomic layer doesn't mean you are done. It doesn't mean the person who you are responding to is finished processing the event. It doesn't mean that they won't continue to grieve, and try to make sense of what happened.

It doesn't mean that in the aftermath of the event they might not have some sleepless nights, engage in deep soul-searching, or decide to change their lives in some way. Brushes with death can re-organize our priorities, they can change us.

I am almost fifty years old. The car accident I just went through, as I study it, taught me something about how easy it is to die. A couple of moments before, I was just a guy driving home from the grocery store, listening to a podcast. The velocity with which my experience went sideways (literally), how quickly this happened (it was no more than three seconds) that the car went from being totally responsive to my steering, to being completely out of control, a mass hurtling through space, is still sobering. The fact that I am alive is a miracle. That there was no one in my blind-spot, that the cars further back were able to stop without hydroplaning, that the person I collided with walked away without serious injury– all of this is miraculous. Thank goodness. But the fact that I was paying attention, didn't do anything wrong, didn't swerve, didn't look away for even a fraction of a second, and still completely lost control of a four thousand pound piece of machinery in a split-second: it is sobering.

And so I continue to examine what that means. Yet the blessing of the autonomic work is that I can contemplate that, study it within myself, examine it, without having my heart race out of control everytime I think of the accident. I can remember and study the event without a residue of arousal. I can get back in a car without feeling nervous. I was able to walk my nervous system back home to itself. And in the places I could not, I was able to lean into a trusted community of support and ask them to help me.

I will probably drive more slowly in the rain now. I will probably be a bit more alert on the highway. I will probably pay attention in a slightly different way, because I have learned something. *But I am not traumatized by the event.*

And, by learning autonomic triage, this is the gift that you can help give to people you serve. You cannot take away the pain of what has happened to them, the emotions they have around it, or what it means. But you can help the animal parts of the body, the wiring of the nervous system that lives at the intersection of spirit and matter to metabolize the energies that it mobilized in order to survive, and in helping someone do this you are giving them a gift that is beyond transaction. There is probably no more valuable gift you can give another person than holding open a door that they can walk through to find their way home.

May you be safe.
May you bring others to safety.

Thank you for your service.

The world needs more people like you
to remind us what it means to be human.

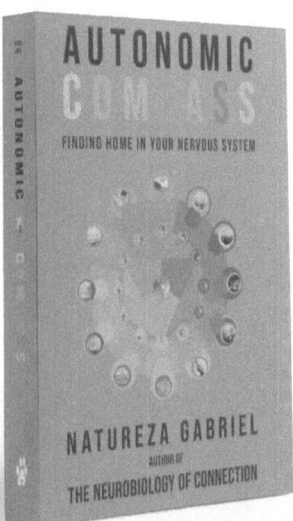

AUTONOMIC COMPASS
FINDING HOME IN YOUR NERVOUS SYSTEM

A clear and practical skills handbook for building autonomic fluency. Learn what the Autonomic Nervous System is, what it does, why it matters, and how to work with it.

Grow your ability to notice, be informed by, and support the needs of your deepest survival systems, which are constantly shaping your interactions with the world.

http://hearthscience.io

ABOUT THE AUTHOR

Natureza Gabriel (aka Gabriel Kram) is the architect of *Autonomics*, a cutting-edge & ancestral update to our understanding of autonomic physiology, which he has developed over 30 years of trans-disciplinary study and research. Gabriel's mind was trained at Yale and Stanford Universities, his heart has been educated in ceremonies and circles. He has spent 30 years studying connection and healing.

He is Founder and CEO of Hearth Science: a translation research firm focused on the deepest drivers of human wellbeing. He is the primary designer of the Autonomic Compass, a proprietary software platform that centralizes autonomic physiology in the diagnosis and treatment of stress-related disorders and the creation of enduring wellbeing. Gabriel is Host and Executive Producer of *The Restorative Practices Film Series, The Connection Masterclass, Evoking Connection States,* and *Lectures on the New Foundation Model in Autonomics*. He has been asked to teach Autonomics to people in 50 countries, executives in Fortune 500 companies, the faculty of medical schools, governments, international NGOs, and tribal leaders. He is the author of the *The Neurobiology of Connection* and twelve other books.

He lives with his family on unceded Miwok territory in Northern California. You can find more of his work, as well as that of the extraordinary faculty of Hearth Science at

HTTP://www.hearthscience.io

www.ingramcontent.com/pod-product-compliance
Lightning Source LLC
Chambersburg PA
CBHW031244120626
46545CB00007B/2637